Copyright

Table of Contents

Introduction

Welcome Message: Establishing empathy and understanding for readers dealing with fear and anxiety.

Personal Note on the Importance of Addressing Fear and Anxiety: Sharing personal experiences or motivations for writing the book.

Chapter 1: Unraveling Fear and Anxiety

Defining Fear and Anxiety: Clarifying the differences and common misconceptions.

Understanding the Physiology of Fear and Anxiety: Exploring the brain's role and the fight-or-flight response.

Common Triggers and Causes: Identifying various triggers and root causes of fear and anxiety.

Chapter 2: The Impact on Mental and Physical Health

Effects of Prolonged Fear and Anxiety: Discussing the impact on mental health, such as increased stress, insomnia, etc.

Relationship between Fear, Anxiety, and Stress: Exploring the interconnectedness and ways to manage stress levels.

Exploring Comorbidities and Associated Conditions: Discussing how fear and anxiety can contribute to or exacerbate other mental health issues.

Chapter 3: Types of Anxiety Disorders

Generalized Anxiety Disorder (GAD): Symptoms, causes, and management strategies.

Panic Disorder: Understanding panic attacks, coping mechanisms, and seeking help.

Social Anxiety Disorder: Strategies for managing social fears and building confidence.

Phobias and Specific Anxiety Triggers: Examining specific fears and methods for overcoming them.

Chapter 4: Coping Mechanisms and Self-Help Strategies

Recognizing and Acknowledging Fear and Anxiety: Encouraging self-awareness and acceptance.

Breathing Techniques and Relaxation Methods: Step-by-step guides for relaxation exercises and their benefits.

Cognitive-Behavioral Strategies for Managing Fear and Anxiety: Practical tips and exercises to challenge negative thought patterns.

Chapter 5: Seeking Professional Help

Importance of Professional Support: Discussing the role of therapists, psychiatrists, and counselors.

Therapy Options: CBT, DBT, Exposure Therapy, etc.: Exploring various therapeutic approaches and their effectiveness.

Medication and Alternative Treatments: Information about medication, holistic approaches, and complementary therapies.

Chapter 6: Lifestyle Changes for Anxiety Management

The Role of Exercise in Reducing Anxiety: Detailing the benefits of exercise and suggesting suitable workout routines.

Nutrition and its Impact on Anxiety Levels: Exploring a balanced diet's influence on mental health.

Sleep Hygiene and its Effect on Mental Well-being: Tips for improving sleep quality and its impact on anxiety.

Chapter 7: Overcoming Specific Fears

Strategies for Overcoming Common Fears: In-depth advice for facing and overcoming specific fears, such as public speaking, fear of failure, etc.

Gradual Exposure Techniques: Step-by-step guides to exposure therapy and desensitization.

Chapter 8: Nurturing Resilience and Building a Support System

Importance of Social Support Networks: Emphasizing the role of friends, family, and community in overcoming fears and anxiety.

Cultivating Resilience in the Face of Fear and Anxiety: Tips for developing mental resilience and emotional strength.

Chapter 9: Mindfulness and Meditation Practices

Incorporating Mindfulness into Daily Life: Techniques for practicing mindfulness in various daily activities.

Guided Meditation Exercises for Anxiety Relief: Audio scripts or step-by-step guides for different meditation practices.

Chapter 10: Moving Forward: Building a Future with Confidence

Setting Realistic Goals for Overcoming Fear and Anxiety: Strategies for setting achievable goals and tracking progress.

Embracing a Life Beyond Fear: Thriving and Flourishing: Encouragement and motivational guidance for a fulfilling life beyond anxiety.

Conclusion

Recap of Key Points: Summarizing the main takeaways from each chapter.

Encouragement and Support for the Reader's Journey: Inspiring final words to motivate readers on their path to overcoming fear and anxiety.

Additional Resources and Support Contacts: Providing a list of further reading materials, hotlines, and support groups for continued assistance.

Introduction

Welcome to "Understanding Fear and Anxiety: Navigating the Path to Inner Peace and Resilience."

Life can be a beautiful journey filled with vibrant colors, but for many of us, there are moments when those colors seem to fade into shades of worry, apprehension, and unease. Fear and anxiety, though natural responses, often overstay their welcome, casting shadows over our experiences and clouding the skies of our well-being.

This book is more than just a collection of words on a page; it's a guiding light, a hand to hold through the labyrinth of emotions. It's a gentle reminder that you are not alone in this journey. Each chapter is crafted with the intention of unraveling the complexities of fear and anxiety, shedding light on their causes, exploring their impacts, and offering a compass to navigate through these challenging terrains.

We start by distinguishing between fear and anxiety, understanding how they manifest, and recognizing the intricate dance between our thoughts and our bodies' responses. Delving deeper, we explore the various types of anxiety disorders, their nuances, and practical strategies to manage them effectively.

This book isn't just about the challenges; it's about solutions. From coping mechanisms and self-help strategies to seeking professional guidance and embracing lifestyle changes, we provide a holistic approach to alleviate and manage fear and anxiety. We offer tools—breathing exercises, mindfulness practices, exposure techniques—to help you reclaim your peace of mind.

Moreover, we emphasize the significance of a support system, encouraging resilience, and setting realistic goals. This journey isn't about eradicating fear entirely, but rather about learning to coexist with it, finding the strength to confront it, and fostering a life that thrives despite its presence.

Throughout this book, you'll find real stories, evidence-based practices, and actionable steps. The aim is not only to inform but to empower you to take control of your mental health, to forge a path toward a life filled with courage, confidence, and a sense of calmness.

Remember, healing is a process, and each step you take is a triumph. Let this book be your companion, guiding you toward a brighter, more resilient version of yourself. You deserve a life where fear and anxiety take a back seat, allowing you to embrace the world with open arms.

Together, let's embark on this journey—a journey toward understanding, acceptance, and ultimately, peace.

Warmly,

Joshua Afolabi.

Chapter 1

Understanding Fear and Anxiety

In the maze of our feelings, not many encounters are basically as multifaceted and unavoidable as dread and tension. They show up excluded, fixing their hold on our psyches, frequently obscuring the lines between the sane and unreasonable, the known and the unexplored world.

Distinguishing Fear from Anxiety

Allow us first to unwind the strings that mesh dread and tension into the texture of our lives. Dread is our body's instinctual reaction to saw dangers. It's that flood of adrenaline when stood up to with impending risk, initiating our instinctive reaction, setting us up to face or dodge what is going on.

Conversely, nervousness waits; a determined concern or disquiet continues past the presence of impending risk. It's the brain's propensity to harp on expected dangers or future vulnerabilities, some of the time with no reasonable beginning or arrangement. A feeling of apprehension, restlessness, or even physical symptoms like a faster heart rate, sweating, and muscle tension are common signs of anxiety.

The Intricacies of Fear and Anxiety

Understanding the complexities of fear and anxiety involves acknowledging their various shades and intensities. Sometimes, fear acts as a protective instinct, guiding us away from harm. However, when fear becomes disproportionate or irrational in response to a perceived threat, it can hinder our daily lives.

Similarly, anxiety, though a natural part of being human, becomes problematic when it disrupts our ability to function. It might lead to avoidance behaviors, negatively impact relationships, or impede our pursuit of personal and professional goals.

The Physiology Behind Fear and Anxiety

The way our brain processes fear and anxiety is very important. Our emotional control center is the amygdala, a structure deep within the brain that looks like an almond. It processes sensory information that comes in and, when it senses a threat, it releases stress hormones to get the body ready for action.

The amygdala also interacts with the prefrontal cortex, which is in charge of rational thought and decision-making. This connection can become distorted during times of increased fear or anxiety, resulting in an amplified emotional response or difficulty controlling it.

Common Triggers and Causes

Dread and uneasiness are complex, emerging from a large number of sources. Horrible encounters, upsetting conditions, hereditary inclinations, or irregular characteristics in mind science can add to their turn of events. Outer factors like cultural tensions, financial vulnerabilities, or critical life altering events can likewise worsen these feelings.

Chapter 2

The Impact on Mental and Physical Health

Despite their intangibility, anxiety and fear have a tangible impact on our mental and physical health. They are not simple passing feelings; rather, they hold the ability to shape our everyday encounters and effect our general wellbeing.

Effects of Prolonged Fear and Anxiety

Drawn out openness to dread and nervousness can significantly affect emotional wellness. Tenacious nervousness might prompt elevated feelings of anxiety, affecting our capacity to focus, decide, and capability successfully in our everyday lives. It can grow into summed up sensations of disquiet, a feeling of looming destruction, or even fits of anxiety, which can be overpowering and crippling.

Furthermore, chronic fear can contribute to the development or exacerbation of mental health conditions such as depression, post-traumatic stress disorder (PTSD), and obsessive-compulsive disorder (OCD). It can also be linked to difficulties in maintaining healthy relationships and can significantly impact self-esteem and confidence.

Relationship between Fear, Anxiety, and Stress
Fear and anxiety are closely entwined with stress, creating a triad that can significantly impact our overall health. Stress is the body's response to any demand or threat, triggering a cascade of physiological reactions. When fear and anxiety persist, the chronic activation of the stress response can lead to detrimental effects on both mental and physical health.

Chronic stress contributes to the wear and tear of the body, affecting the immune system, cardiovascular health, and even accelerating the aging process. Moreover, the perpetual activation of stress hormones can impair memory, disrupt sleep patterns, and exacerbate existing health conditions.

Exploring Comorbidities and Associated Conditions
Fear and anxiety seldom walk alone; they often coexist with other mental health conditions or contribute to their development. For instance, individuals grappling with anxiety disorders might also experience substance abuse, eating disorders, or chronic pain conditions.

Moreover, fear and anxiety can manifest in physical symptoms, such as tension headaches, gastrointestinal issues, or exacerbation of pre-existing conditions like asthma or heart disease. Addressing mental health concerns becomes imperative not only for emotional well-being but also for the holistic maintenance of physical health.
Understanding the profound impact of fear and anxiety on both mental and physical health underscores the urgency of addressing these emotions. The interplay between our mental state and physical well-being necessitates a comprehensive approach to effectively manage and mitigate the adverse effects of these emotions.

Chapter 3

Types of Anxiety Disorders

Fear and anxiety manifest in various forms, each with its nuances and impacts on our lives. Understanding the specific characteristics of different anxiety disorders is pivotal in recognizing, addressing, and managing these complex emotions.

Generalized Anxiety Disorder (GAD)

Generalized Anxiety Disorder is marked by excessive worry and apprehension about various aspects of life, often without a specific trigger or reason. Individuals with GAD experience persistent and uncontrollable concerns about everyday occurrences, such as health, work, relationships, and finances. These worries often lead to physical symptoms like restlessness, irritability, muscle tension, and difficulty concentrating.

Panic Disorder

Panic Disorder involves recurrent and unexpected panic attacks, which are intense surges of fear or discomfort that reach a peak within minutes. These attacks can be accompanied by palpitations, sweating, trembling, shortness of breath, and a sense of impending doom or loss of control. Fear of future panic attacks can lead to changes in behavior and avoidance of places or situations where attacks have occurred previously.

Social Anxiety Disorder

Social Anxiety Disorder, also known as social phobia, revolves around an intense fear of social situations where individuals feel scrutinized, judged, or embarrassed. It goes beyond mere shyness and can significantly impact one's ability to engage in social interactions or perform in public settings. Fear of being negatively evaluated by others can lead to avoidance behaviors, isolation, and hindrance in personal and professional growth.

Phobias and Specific Anxiety Triggers

Phobias entail an overwhelming fear of specific objects, situations, or activities. These fears are excessive and unreasonable, often leading to intense anxiety or panic when confronted with the particular phobic stimulus. Common phobias include fear of heights (acrophobia), fear of flying (aviophobia), fear of enclosed spaces (claustrophobia), or fear of animals (zoophobia). Phobias can significantly disrupt daily life if left unaddressed.

Understanding the nuances of these anxiety disorders is the first step toward effective management and seeking appropriate help. Identifying specific symptoms and patterns within these disorders can guide individuals toward suitable treatments and coping strategies tailored to their needs.

Chapter 4

Coping Mechanisms and Self-Help Strategies

Fear and anxiety, while daunting, are not insurmountable. Equipping ourselves with coping mechanisms and self-help strategies empowers us to navigate through the labyrinth of these emotions and reclaim our sense of calmness and control.

Recognizing and Acknowledging Fear and Anxiety

Acknowledgment is the first step toward managing fear and anxiety. It involves recognizing and accepting these emotions without judgment. By acknowledging their presence, we pave the way for self-awareness and understanding, creating a foundation for effective coping strategies.

Breathing Techniques and Relaxation Methods

Our breath is an anchor in turbulent seas. Utilizing breathing techniques and relaxation methods can be immensely beneficial in calming the mind and alleviating anxiety. Techniques such as deep breathing, progressive muscle relaxation, and guided imagery help in grounding oneself and reducing the intensity of anxious feelings.

Cognitive-Behavioral Strategies for Managing Fear and Anxiety

Cognitive-behavioral strategies focus on identifying and challenging negative thought patterns associated with fear and anxiety. By examining and restructuring our thoughts, we can alter our emotional responses. Techniques like cognitive restructuring, thought stopping, and reframing help in replacing anxious thoughts with more rational and balanced perspectives.

Mindfulness and Meditation Practices

Mindfulness practices cultivate a heightened awareness of the present moment, fostering a non-judgmental acceptance of our thoughts and emotions. Mindfulness-based techniques, meditation, and mindfulness exercises enable us to observe our feelings without getting entangled in them. Through consistent practice, individuals can develop resilience against anxiety triggers.

Self-Care Routines and Stress Management

Self-care plays a pivotal role in managing fear and anxiety. Engaging in activities that nurture the mind and body—such as regular exercise, adequate sleep, maintaining a healthy diet, and engaging in hobbies—helps in reducing stress levels and enhancing overall well-being.

Seeking Support and Building Coping Strategies

Exploring support systems, whether through trusted friends, family, or support groups, can offer solace and understanding during difficult times. Additionally, building a toolkit of coping strategies that resonate personally—such as journaling, creative expression, or relaxation exercises—empowers individuals to confront and manage anxiety effectively.

Embracing a Multifaceted Approach

Combining these coping mechanisms and self-help strategies allows for a multifaceted approach to managing fear and anxiety. Each individual may find certain techniques more effective than others, emphasizing the importance of exploring and customizing a repertoire of strategies that suit one's preferences and needs.

Chapter 5

Seeking Professional Help

Fear and anxiety can at times become overwhelming, affecting various aspects of our lives. Seeking professional guidance and support can be a crucial step in managing these emotions and reclaiming our mental well-being.
Importance of Professional Support
Professional help offers specialized guidance from mental health practitioners trained in addressing anxiety disorders and related issues. Seeking assistance is

not a sign of weakness but a courageous step toward understanding and managing these complex emotions.

Therapy Options: CBT, DBT, Exposure Therapy, etc.
Various therapeutic approaches are available to address fear and anxiety. Cognitive-Behavioral Therapy (CBT) focuses on identifying and modifying negative thought patterns and behaviors. Dialectical Behavior Therapy (DBT) emphasizes mindfulness, emotion regulation, and interpersonal effectiveness. Exposure Therapy involves gradual exposure to feared situations to reduce anxiety responses.

Medication and Alternative Treatments
In some cases, medication may be prescribed by healthcare professionals to alleviate the symptoms of anxiety disorders. Anti-anxiety medications, antidepressants, and beta-blockers are among the options available.

Additionally, alternative treatments like acupuncture, yoga, aromatherapy, or herbal supplements are explored by some individuals for anxiety management.

Collaborative Treatment Approaches
Effective treatment often involves a collaborative approach between mental health professionals, individuals seeking help, and their support systems. Creating a treatment plan tailored to the individual's needs and preferences enhances the effectiveness of therapy and fosters a supportive environment for recovery.

Overcoming Barriers to Seeking Help
Several barriers, such as stigma, financial constraints, or lack of accessibility, may hinder individuals from seeking professional help. Addressing these barriers by raising awareness, exploring affordable options, utilizing teletherapy services, or seeking community support can facilitate access to mental health care.

Importance of Consistency and Patience
Recovery from fear and anxiety is a process that requires time, commitment, and patience. It's essential to attend therapy sessions regularly, actively participate in treatment, and communicate openly with healthcare providers. Overcoming these emotions is a journey that necessitates perseverance and dedication.

Empowerment through Professional Guidance
Professional help empowers individuals by equipping them with coping strategies, offering insights into their emotions, and providing a safe space to

address fears and anxieties. It facilitates a deeper understanding of oneself and fosters resilience to navigate life's challenges.

Chapter 6

Lifestyle Changes for Anxiety Management

The intertwining relationship between our lifestyle choices and our mental well-being cannot be overstated. Making deliberate lifestyle changes can significantly impact our ability to manage and alleviate anxiety.

The Role of Exercise in Reducing Anxiety

Physical activity has proven to be a powerful tool in managing anxiety. Regular exercise helps in reducing stress hormones, increasing the production of endorphins (the body's natural mood elevators), and promoting relaxation. Engaging in activities like yoga, running, swimming, or simply taking walks can effectively alleviate symptoms of anxiety.

Nutrition and its Impact on Anxiety Levels

Maintaining a balanced and nutritious diet is crucial for mental health. Certain foods and nutrients play a role in regulating mood and anxiety levels.

Consuming omega-3 fatty acids, complex carbohydrates, antioxidants, and foods rich in magnesium and zinc can positively influence anxiety. Conversely, minimizing caffeine, refined sugars, and processed foods may help in reducing anxiety symptoms.

Sleep Hygiene and its Effect on Mental Well-being

Quality sleep is essential for emotional regulation and mental clarity. Establishing a consistent sleep schedule, creating a relaxing bedtime routine, and ensuring a comfortable sleep environment are key components of good sleep hygiene. Lack of sleep can exacerbate anxiety symptoms, making it imperative to prioritize adequate rest for optimal mental health.

Stress Management Techniques

Developing stress management techniques is pivotal in mitigating anxiety. Practicing mindfulness, deep breathing exercises, or engaging in activities like journaling, art therapy, or listening to calming music can help in reducing stress levels. Additionally, incorporating relaxation techniques such as progressive muscle relaxation or guided imagery aids in calming the mind and body.

Balancing Work and Leisure

Maintaining a healthy work-life balance is crucial for managing anxiety. Setting boundaries, taking regular breaks, and engaging in leisure activities or hobbies that bring joy and relaxation foster a sense of fulfillment and reduce stress. Allocating time for oneself and cultivating interests outside of work can significantly contribute to mental well-being.

Holistic Approach to Self-Care

Adopting a holistic approach to self-care—addressing physical, emotional, and social needs—promotes overall mental health. Engaging in activities that nurture the mind, body, and spirit, such as meditation, spending time in nature, practicing gratitude, or fostering social connections, enhances resilience and aids in anxiety management.

The Power of Lifestyle Modifications

Embracing lifestyle changes serves as a potent complement to other anxiety management strategies. Small, intentional adjustments in daily routines can yield profound improvements in mental well-being. Cultivating a lifestyle that supports emotional health is instrumental in managing anxiety and fostering a sense of balance and calmness.

Chapter 7

Overcoming Specific Fears

Fear often manifests itself in specific forms, presenting unique challenges to those who grapple with them. Understanding strategies to confront and overcome these specific fears empowers individuals to reclaim control over their lives.

Strategies for Overcoming Common Fears

Fear of Public Speaking: Gradual exposure, practice, and visualization techniques can help in desensitizing the fear of public speaking. Joining public speaking groups or seeking professional guidance enables individuals to build confidence and improve communication skills.

Fear of Failure: Reframing perspectives on failure as opportunities for growth and learning assists in overcoming the fear of failure. Setting realistic goals, accepting imperfections, and celebrating small achievements foster resilience in the face of setbacks.

Fear of Heights (Acrophobia): Exposure therapy, progressive desensitization, and relaxation techniques aid in overcoming the fear of heights. Slowly confronting height-related situations in a controlled and supportive environment helps in reducing anxiety responses.

Fear of Flying (Aviophobia): Education about airplane safety, gradual exposure to flight-related scenarios, and relaxation techniques assist in managing the fear of flying. Seeking support from flight anxiety programs or therapy can help in addressing and managing flight-related fears.

Fear of Enclosed Spaces (Claustrophobia): Controlled exposure to confined spaces, practicing relaxation techniques, and gradual desensitization assist in overcoming claustrophobia. Learning coping strategies to manage anxiety during situations involving enclosed spaces is pivotal for progress.

Gradual Exposure Techniques
Gradual exposure involves systematically and gradually confronting feared situations or objects in a controlled manner. By exposing oneself to incremental levels of anxiety-provoking stimuli, individuals learn to manage and ultimately reduce their fear response. This method, practiced under professional guidance, helps in building confidence and reducing anxiety triggers.

Building Confidence through Successive Triumphs
Successive triumphs over specific fears reinforce confidence and resilience. Celebrating small victories, even if they seem insignificant, contributes to a sense of accomplishment and aids in gradual desensitization. Consistent effort and perseverance pave the way toward overcoming specific fears.

Embracing Support and Professional Guidance
Seeking support from friends, family, or support groups while confronting specific fears provides encouragement and a sense of solidarity. Professional guidance from therapists or counselors trained in treating specific phobias offers structured approaches tailored to individual needs.

The Journey to Overcoming Specific Fears
Overcoming specific fears is a journey marked by dedication, patience, and courage. Understanding and confronting these fears head-on, employing various strategies, and seeking professional assistance when needed pave the path toward liberation from their grip.

Chapter 8

Nurturing Resilience and Building a Support System

In the face of fear and anxiety, fostering resilience and cultivating a robust support system serve as pillars of strength, offering invaluable resources for navigating life's challenges.

Importance of Social Support Networks

Establishing and maintaining social connections play a pivotal role in managing fear and anxiety. Supportive relationships with friends, family, or community groups offer empathy, understanding, and a sense of belonging. Sharing experiences and feelings with trusted individuals can alleviate emotional distress and reduce the sense of isolation.

Cultivating Resilience in the Face of Fear and Anxiety

Resilience is the ability to adapt and bounce back from adversity. Cultivating resilience involves developing coping skills, fostering a positive outlook, and maintaining a sense of purpose. Embracing challenges as opportunities for growth, practicing self-compassion, and learning from setbacks are integral components of resilience-building.

Embracing Positive Coping Mechanisms

Positive coping mechanisms bolster resilience and aid in managing anxiety. Engaging in activities that promote emotional well-being—such as practicing gratitude, maintaining optimism, nurturing a sense of humor, or finding purpose in hobbies or volunteer work—contributes to emotional resilience and buffers against stress.

Seeking Professional Support for Resilience Building

Therapists or counselors proficient in building resilience can offer guidance and tools to enhance one's ability to cope with fear and anxiety. Therapeutic approaches focusing on resilience-building, cognitive restructuring, and stress management equip individuals with skills to navigate adversity effectively.

The Role of Mindset in Resilience

Mindset shapes our responses to challenges. Adopting a growth mindset—viewing setbacks as opportunities for learning and growth—fosters resilience. Recognizing and reframing negative thought patterns into more adaptive ones facilitates resilience in the face of fear and anxiety.

Building a Support System for Long-Term Well-being

Constructing a robust support system involves fostering connections, both within oneself and with others. Prioritizing self-care, nurturing healthy relationships, seeking professional guidance when needed, and participating in support groups or community activities contribute to a comprehensive support network.

Empowerment through Resilience and Support

Resilience and a strong support system empower individuals to navigate through fear and anxiety with strength and determination. Recognizing one's ability to adapt, grow, and seek assistance when necessary fosters a sense of empowerment and resilience in facing life's challenges.

Chapter 9

Mindfulness and Meditation Practices

In the pursuit of managing fear and anxiety, the practice of mindfulness and meditation emerges as a powerful tool, offering a sanctuary amidst the chaos of our thoughts and emotions.

Incorporating Mindfulness into Daily Life

Mindfulness involves cultivating a heightened awareness and attention to the present moment without judgment. Integrating mindfulness into daily life activities—such as mindful eating, walking, or even engaging in routine tasks—promotes a sense of calmness and clarity. By anchoring our attention to the present, we can reduce anxiety related to past regrets or future uncertainties.

Techniques for Practicing Mindfulness

Mindfulness practices encompass a variety of techniques. Mindful breathing exercises, body scan meditations, and focused attention on sensory experiences help in grounding oneself in the present moment. These techniques allow individuals to observe thoughts and emotions without getting entangled in them, fostering a sense of detachment and inner peace.

Guided Meditation Exercises for Anxiety Relief

Guided meditation sessions offer structured exercises led by an instructor or through audio recordings. These sessions guide individuals through relaxation techniques, visualization exercises, or body-centered meditations aimed at alleviating anxiety. Guided meditations for anxiety often focus on deep relaxation and cultivating a sense of tranquility.

The Benefits of Mindfulness and Meditation

Scientific research supports the multitude of benefits derived from mindfulness and meditation practices. These include reduced stress levels, improved emotional regulation, enhanced focus and concentration, better sleep quality, and an overall sense of well-being. Regular practice of mindfulness has shown to rewire the brain, promoting resilience against anxiety triggers.

Incorporating Mindfulness into Anxiety Management

Mindfulness serves as a powerful ally in managing anxiety. By observing thoughts and emotions with curiosity rather than judgment, individuals develop a sense of detachment from anxiety-provoking stimuli. Mindfulness enables individuals to respond to anxiety with greater clarity and resilience, reducing the grip that fear and worry may hold.

Making Mindfulness a Daily Practice

Consistency is key in reaping the benefits of mindfulness and meditation. Establishing a regular practice, even if for a few minutes each day, fosters the integration of mindfulness into one's lifestyle. Whether through guided sessions, smartphone apps, or formal training, making mindfulness a habit amplifies its impact on anxiety management.

Embracing the Calmness Within

Mindfulness and meditation practices offer a sanctuary—a refuge amidst the storm of anxious thoughts and emotions. By cultivating a moment-to-moment awareness and allowing space for tranquility within, individuals develop resilience and find solace in the midst of life's challenges.

Chapter 10

Moving Forward: Building a Future with Confidence

Amidst the complexities of fear and anxiety, lies the possibility of transcending these emotions and embracing a life brimming with courage, resilience, and fulfillment. Moving forward involves a deliberate journey toward self-empowerment and growth.

Setting Realistic Goals for Overcoming Fear and Anxiety
Setting achievable goals marks the beginning of a path toward overcoming fear and anxiety. Establishing specific, measurable, and realistic goals provides direction and motivation. Incremental progress toward these goals—no matter how small—serves as a testament to resilience and determination.

Embracing a Comprehensive Approach to Well-being
Recognizing that emotional well-being is a culmination of various factors encourages a holistic approach. Balancing physical health, mental wellness, social connections, and self-care activities forms a solid foundation for a fulfilling life beyond anxiety.

Embracing a Life Beyond Fear
Thriving and flourishing despite the presence of fear involves a shift in perspective. It's about accepting fear as a part of the human experience rather than allowing it to define life. Embracing uncertainties, taking calculated risks, and cultivating a growth-oriented mindset propel individuals toward a life enriched with possibilities.

Nurturing Resilience in the Face of Challenges
Challenges are an inevitable part of life's tapestry. Nurturing resilience equips individuals with the tools to face adversity with strength and adaptability. Learning from setbacks, practicing self-compassion, and acknowledging personal growth amid challenges foster resilience.

Celebrating Progress and Small Victories
Amidst the journey of managing fear and anxiety, it's crucial to acknowledge and celebrate progress. Recognizing even the smallest steps toward growth and well-being cultivates a positive outlook and reinforces the courage needed to confront fears.

Embracing a Growth Mindset
Adopting a growth mindset emphasizes the potential for growth and development. Viewing failures as opportunities for learning, embracing change, and seeking new experiences instills a sense of resilience and curiosity about life's possibilities.

Fostering a Future with Confidence
Confidence emerges from a deep understanding of oneself, acceptance of vulnerabilities, and an unwavering belief in one's abilities. Cultivating self-confidence involves embracing authenticity, trusting one's intuition, and valuing personal strengths.

Thriving Beyond Fear and Anxiety

Thriving beyond fear and anxiety is not merely about conquering these emotions but about thriving despite their presence. It's about weaving a life rich in meaning, purpose, and fulfillment—a life that transcends the limitations imposed by fear.

Conclusion

Embracing a Life Beyond Fear and Anxiety

As this transformative journey through understanding fear and anxiety culminates, it becomes evident that the pursuit of a life unencumbered by fear isn't about eradicating these emotions entirely. Instead, it's a voyage toward coexistence, resilience, and a profound sense of empowerment.

The journey we've embarked upon is not a finite destination but rather a continuous evolution—a process of learning, unlearning, and redefining our relationship with fear and anxiety. It's about acknowledging their presence without allowing them to dictate the course of our lives.

Each chapter has unraveled layers, providing insights, strategies, and tools to navigate the intricate maze of emotions. We've explored the intricate workings of fear and anxiety, dissected their impact on mental and physical health, and delved into coping mechanisms and support systems.

Moving forward involves setting sail toward a future brimming with confidence and resilience. It's about setting realistic goals, nurturing resilience, and celebrating the triumphs—no matter how small. It's acknowledging the progress made, embodying self-compassion, and embracing a growth-oriented mindset.

Confidence doesn't spring from the absence of fear but from the courage to confront it. It emanates from self-awareness, self-acceptance, and an unwavering belief in our capacity to overcome challenges. Confidence blooms when we recognize our strengths and bravely embrace our vulnerabilities.

Thriving beyond fear and anxiety doesn't signify an absence of these emotions; rather, it's about thriving despite their presence. It's about weaving a life rich in purpose, authenticity, and meaning—a life that embraces challenges as opportunities for growth and transformation.

As you continue on your journey, remember that every step you take, every effort you make to confront fear and anxiety, is a testament to your courage. Embrace the resilience you've cultivated, celebrate the progress you've made, and be compassionate with yourself in moments of difficulty.

You possess within you an inherent strength—a strength that enables you to navigate the ebb and flow of life's uncertainties. You are capable of crafting a narrative that transcends fear, embraces resilience, and thrives in the face of adversity.

So, as you venture forth, carry with you the wisdom gleaned from this journey. Embrace the challenges, celebrate the victories, and live a life rooted in courage, authenticity, and boundless resilience.

Remember, your story is still being written. Embrace it with courage, grace, and the unwavering belief that within you lies the power to shape a life beyond fear—a life filled with boundless possibilities.

www.ingramcontent.com/pod-product-compliance
Lightning Source LLC
Chambersburg PA
CBHW080924260726
48661CB00009B/3791